THRIVING BEYOND

40

How To Achieve Optimal Health And Wellness For A Fulfilling Life

J.C. OSORIO

Table of Contents

Disclaimer

The information provided in this book is for general informational purposes only. While every effort has been made to ensure the accuracy and completeness of the information presented, the author and publisher make no representations or warranties of any kind, express or implied, about the suitability, reliability, or applicability of the content for any specific individual or purpose.

The content of this book is not intended to be a substitute for professional medical advice, diagnosis, or treatment. Always seek the advice of a qualified healthcare provider with any questions you may have regarding a medical condition or before embarking on any exercise or dietary program.

The author and publisher of this book are not responsible for any adverse effects or consequences resulting from the use of the information presented herein. Any reliance you place on the information within this book is strictly at your own risk.

The inclusion of any third-party resources, websites, or references does not imply endorsement or recommendation by the author and publisher. The author and publisher shall have no responsibility for the content, accuracy, or availability of external sites or resources mentioned in this book.

The testimonials and success stories shared in this book are based on individual experiences, and results may vary. The author and publisher do not guarantee any specific outcomes or results from implementing the suggestions and recommendations provided in this book.

It is important to consult with a qualified professional, such as a healthcare provider or fitness expert, before making any significant changes to your lifestyle, exercise routine, or diet.

By reading this book, you acknowledge and agree that the author and publisher are not liable for any direct or indirect damages or losses arising from the use of the information contained herein.

Every individual is unique, and what works for one person may not work for another. It is essential to listen to your body, respect your limits, and make informed decisions based on your specific circumstances.

The information presented in this book is subject to change and may not be up to date at the time of your reading. The author and publisher do not assume any responsibility or liability for any errors or omissions that may occur.

In conclusion, the information provided in this book is intended to inspire and educate, but it should not replace personalized advice or professional guidance. It is recommended to consult with appropriate experts and professionals for specific concerns and circumstances

Introduction

Welcome to "Thriving Beyond 40: How to Achieve Optimal Health and Wellness for a Fulfilling Life." This book is a heartfelt guide that will empower you to take charge of your health, embrace positive changes, and embark on a transformative journey towards a vibrant life, even after reaching the milestone of 40.

In a world where the narrative around aging is often negative and limiting, this book aims to shatter those misconceptions and inspire you to rewrite your own story. It draws inspiration from scientific research, real-life success stories, and lessons learned from renowned health and wellness experts.

I have witnessed countless individuals in their 40s and beyond transform their lives by making conscious choices and taking dedicated action. Through this book, I aim to share their wisdom, along with evidence-based strategies, to help you unlock your full potential and embrace a life of vitality, purpose, and fulfillment.

Each chapter will guide you step-by-step, offering practical advice, insightful anecdotes, and actionable tips. I encourage you to take notes and reflect on your own experiences as you progress through this emotional and motivating journey. At the end of each chapter, you'll find action items that will propel you toward positive change.

Together, let's challenge societal norms, break free from limiting beliefs, and redefine what it means to age gracefully. Are you ready to embark on this extraordinary path towards being in the best shape of your life and experiencing a healthy life after 40? Let's begin!

Dedication

Dedicated to my Dad, The best person I have ever known.

Thank you for all the love you always gave to me and your Family.

I love you and miss you a lot!

Embracing the Journey:

A New Beginning at 40

In the twilight of your 30s, you stand at the crossroads of life. The milestone of 40 is fast approaching, and with it comes a mixture of emotions - anticipation, reflection, and perhaps a tinge of apprehension. But let me assure you, my friend, that this is not the end of youth or the beginning of decline. Instead, it marks the dawn of a new chapter, an opportunity to embrace life with renewed vigor and embark on a journey toward the best version of yourself.

As the clock strikes midnight on your 40th birthday, take a moment to honor the path you've traveled so far. Celebrate the wisdom gained from the lessons life has bestowed upon you. Every triumph and setback, every laughter and tear, has molded you into the resilient soul you are today. You've weathered storms and emerged stronger, wiser, and more determined than ever before.

Now, as you turn the page to this new chapter, it's time to rewrite the narrative. Let go of the societal expectations that label 40 as a time of decline, and instead, embrace the limitless possibilities that lie ahead. This is your moment to reclaim your health, rediscover your passions, and reignite the fire within your soul.

But how do you ask? The answer lies in understanding the true nature of aging. It's not a linear descent into frailty and disarray. No, my friend, it's a complex tapestry woven by the interplay of your lifestyle choices, genetics, and mindset. You hold the brush, and it's time to paint a vibrant masterpiece.

In the chapters that follow, we will delve deep into the science of aging, exploring the intricacies of cellular renewal, hormonal balance, and the remarkable resilience of the human body. We will debunk the myths surrounding aging and arm you with the knowledge needed to make informed choices.

Remember, you are not alone on this journey. Draw inspiration from those who have paved the way for us. The authors of "Younger Next Year" and "The Blue Zones" have illuminated the path to vitality and longevity. They have shown us that age is just a number and that with the right mindset, lifestyle modifications, and a supportive community, we can thrive well into our golden years.

But this is more than just a physical transformation. It's about nourishing your mind, body, and soul. It's about finding balance in an imbalanced world and cultivating a sense of inner peace. It's about embracing self-care, not as an indulgence, but as a vital component of a life well-lived.

As we embark on this emotional journey together, I urge you to approach each chapter with an open heart and a willingness to challenge the status quo. Take notes, reflect on your own experiences, and most importantly, take action. True transformation happens not in the pages of a book but in the choices you make each day.

At the end of this book, I promise you'll emerge with a newfound sense of purpose, armed with practical tools to achieve optimal health, and a soul on fire with the passion for life. So, my friend, let's take the first step together and embrace the journey that awaits us. The best years of your life are yet to come.

Turn the page, and let the adventure begin.

Unveiling the Aging Process: Understanding the Science of Aging

As we dive into the second chapter of our journey, let us embark on a voyage of discovery—a quest to unravel the mysteries of the aging process. Understanding the science behind aging is the key to unlocking the door to vibrant health and vitality.

At its core, aging is a natural phenomenon—a beautifully intricate dance between our genetic makeup and the environment we inhabit. Our bodies are composed of trillions of cells, each with its unique role and purpose. Over time, however, the wear and tear of daily life, along with a myriad of other factors, can take a toll on these tiny building blocks of life.

But fear not, for within the depths of our DNA lies the remarkable ability to repair and rejuvenate. It's a delicate balance, a constant battle between damage and regeneration, and our lifestyle choices play a pivotal role in tipping the scales in favor of youthfulness and vitality.

Imagine your body as a finely tuned instrument, a symphony waiting to be conducted. Every note, every rhythm is orchestrated by the delicate interplay of hormones, neurotransmitters, and cellular communication. When this symphony is in harmony, we experience optimal health, boundless energy, and a radiant glow. But when discordant notes emerge, we may find ourselves out of tune, struggling to maintain our well-being.

In this chapter, we will delve into the fascinating world of hormones—chemical messengers that dictate the tempo of our existence. Hormones are the maestros of our bodies, influencing our metabolism, mood, sleep, and countless other bodily functions. Understanding the delicate balance of these hormonal symphonies is key to unlocking the secrets of vitality.

We will explore the profound impact of lifestyle choices on hormone production and regulation. Nutrition, exercise, sleep, and stress management—they all play critical roles in nurturing hormonal harmony. By making intentional choices in these areas, we can create a harmonious symphony within, leading to a life filled with boundless energy and a sense of well-being.

But the journey doesn't end with hormones alone. We must also venture into the realms of cellular rejuvenation and the fascinating world of telomeres. These protective caps at the ends of our chromosomes play a crucial role in determining our biological age. Through the intricate dance of lifestyle choices, we can protect and even lengthen our telomeres, slowing down the aging process and defying the limits of time.

Now, dear reader, it's time to take a deep breath and immerse yourself in the wonders of scientific discovery. As we journey through this chapter together, let the emotions stir within you. Feel the awe and wonder that comes from understanding the delicate intricacies of your being. Take notes, ask questions, and most importantly, let this newfound knowledge inspire you to take action.

At the end of this chapter, you'll find action items that will guide you on your path to vibrant aging. Remember, this journey is not a sprint but a marathon—a lifelong commitment to nurturing your body, mind, and soul. So, let us dive into the depths of the aging process, armed with knowledge, curiosity, and an unwavering belief in our ability to shape our destinies.

The symphony awaits. It's time to conduct the melody of your life and embrace the science of aging with open arms. Together, let us rewrite the script of our lives and embark on a journey toward timeless vitality.

Actions to Take: Symphony of Life

1. Embrace the Melody Within Today, and take a moment to appreciate the exquisite symphony playing within your body. Listen closely to the intricate notes of hormones, neurotransmitters, and cellular communication. Feel the rhythm of life pulsating through your veins. Let this awareness ignite a deep sense of gratitude for the miracle that is you.

2. Tune Your Lifestyle Choices: Just as a conductor fine-tunes an orchestra, you have the power to shape your symphony. Nourish your body with vibrant whole foods.

3. Engage in joyful movement that invigorates your spirit. Prioritize restful sleep and cultivate healthy stress management practices. By making conscious choices, you harmonize the elements of your life, creating a melody that resonates with vitality.

4. Unveil the Secrets of Hormonal Harmony: Dive into the fascinating world of hormones and their impact on your well-being. Educate yourself on the profound connection between nutrition, exercise, and hormone regulation. Choose foods that support hormone balance, engage in physical activities that boost their production, and revel in the positive effects on your mood, energy, and overall vitality.

5. Protect Your Telomeres, Preserve Your Youth: Explore the captivating science of telomeres, those guardians of youthfulness at the ends of your chromosomes. With every lifestyle choice you make, remember that you hold the power to protect and lengthen these precious caps. Nurture your telomeres with healthy habits, such as meditation, stress reduction, and antioxidant-rich nutrition. By doing so, you unlock the potential for a longer, more vibrant life.

6. Feel the Awe of Scientific Discovery: Allow yourself to be captivated by the wonders of the aging process unfolding before you. Let the emotions of awe and wonder fill your heart as you delve deeper into the mysteries of your being. Recognize that you are part of a vast, interconnected web of life and that by understanding the science behind aging, you are embarking on a journey of self-empowerment and transformation.

7. Take Inspired Notes: As you absorb the knowledge shared in this chapter, grab a pen and paper. Jot down the insights and revelations that resonate deeply with you. Write down your questions and curiosities, allowing them to fuel your thirst for knowledge. By documenting your thoughts, you create a tangible reminder of your commitment to growth and transformation.

8. Ask Bold Questions: Don't be afraid to challenge the status quo. Engage in conversations, seek out experts, and explore alternative perspectives. Ask thought-provoking questions that challenge conventional wisdom. By doing so, you

become an active participant in the ongoing dialogue about aging, and your inquiries pave the way for innovative solutions and discoveries.

9. Commit to Lifelong Learning: Remember, the journey toward vibrant aging is not a destination but a continuous expedition. Commit to a lifelong pursuit of knowledge and growth. Stay abreast of scientific advancements, and immerse yourself in books, podcasts, and seminars that expand your understanding. Embrace the mindset of a lifelong learner, and let the pursuit of wisdom be the fuel that propels you forward.

10. Share Your Symphony: Your journey toward timeless vitality is not meant to be traveled alone. Share your knowledge, experiences, and inspiration with others. Be a beacon of light, guiding those around you toward their paths of vibrant aging. By uplifting and supporting others on their journeys, you create a symphony of collective well-being that reverberates far beyond your own life.

MY NOTES:

C h a p t e r   3

Igniting the Flame Within:

Cultivating a Positive Mindset for Success

Dear reader, as we venture into the realms of the third chapter, let us delve into the transformative power of the mind—a force that can ignite the flame within and propel us toward a life of boundless possibilities. It is said that the mind is both a battleground and a sanctuary, capable of shaping our reality and determining the trajectory of our lives.

At the heart of it, all lies the power of mindset—a catalyst for change, a source of resilience, and a beacon of hope. It is within our minds that dreams are born, challenges are conquered, and our true potential is unleashed. It is here that the seeds of motivation, determination, and belief take root, blossoming into a life that surpasses all expectations.

But the mind, like a delicate flower, requires nurturing and cultivation. It is all too easy to fall into the traps of self-doubt, negativity, and limiting beliefs. The world may throw obstacles in our path, and our inner critic may whisper words of defeat. Yet, it is in these moments that we must rise above, embracing the power of a positive mindset.

In this chapter, we will explore the profound impact of our thoughts, beliefs, and self-talk on our overall well-being. We will learn how to harness the power of affirmations, visualization, and gratitude to create a fertile ground for growth. By rewiring our minds, we can transform our lives from within.

Let me be clear, dear reader, cultivating a positive mindset does not mean denying the realities of life or living in a state of perpetual bliss. It is about acknowledging the challenges we face while embracing the power to overcome them. It is about finding strength in vulnerability, resilience in the face of adversity, and gratitude amidst the chaos.

We will draw inspiration from the wisdom of renowned psychologists, spiritual teachers, and motivational speakers who have illuminated the path to emotional well-being. Their teachings remind us that we have the power to shape our narratives, rewrite the stories that hold us back, and embrace a life of purpose, passion, and joy.

Throughout this chapter, you will find practical exercises and techniques that will empower you to nurture a positive mindset. Take the time to reflect, journal your thoughts, and explore the depths of your inner world. Let your emotions flow freely as you uncover the layers of conditioning that may have hindered your growth.

Remember, dear reader, you are worthy of a life filled with happiness, abundance, and fulfillment. The flame within you is waiting to be ignited, and it is through the power of a positive mindset that you can fan the flames and set your life ablaze with passion and purpose.

As we journey through this emotional chapter, allow yourself to feel the surge of inspiration, the flicker of hope, and the realization that you have the power to create a life that transcends the ordinary. With each step forward, you will be closer to embracing the best shape of your life and experiencing the richness that comes from a healthy life after 40.

So, let us embark on this transformative quest, together hand in hand, as we cultivate a positive mindset that will illuminate our path and guide us towards a life of extraordinary possibilities. The power is within you. Let it shine, and let us create a symphony of resilience, optimism, and unwavering belief in our ability to thrive beyond measure.

Actions to Take: Ignite the Flame Within

1. Embrace the Power of Mindset: Today, make a conscious decision to embrace the immense power of your mindset. Recognize that your thoughts, beliefs, and self-talk shape your reality. Choose to believe in your potential, to see opportunities where others see obstacles, and to cultivate a positive outlook on life. Let this shift in perspective be the spark that ignites the flame within you.

2. Rewrite Your Inner Narrative: Take a pen and paper, and begin to rewrite the stories you tell yourself. Challenge the limiting beliefs that have held you back and replace them with empowering narratives of resilience and possibility. Allow yourself to envision a future where you are thriving, achieving your dreams, and living a life filled with purpose. Let this new narrative become the guiding light on your path to success.

3. Nurture Daily Affirmations: Integrate the practice of affirmations into your daily routine. Choose empowering statements that resonate with you, such as "I am capable of overcoming any challenge" or "I attract abundance and positivity into my life." Repeat these affirmations with conviction, allowing them to permeate your subconscious mind and shape your reality. Feel the emotions they evoke and let them fuel your actions.

4. Visualize Your Ideal Future: Close your eyes and visualize the life you desire. See yourself accomplishing your goals, experiencing joy, and living with purpose. Engage all your senses in this visualization—feel the excitement, taste the victory, and hear the applause. Immerse yourself in the emotions of success and let them guide your actions in the present moment. Visualize yourself as the person you aspire to be, and watch the flame within grow brighter.

5. Practice Gratitude: Cultivate a daily practice of gratitude. Take a few moments each day to reflect on the blessings in your life, both big and small. Write down three things you are grateful for and truly savor the emotions that arise. Gratitude shifts your focus from what is lacking to what is abundant, opening your heart to joy and appreciation. Let gratitude become the foundation for a positive mindset that attracts more reasons to be grateful.

6. Surround Yourself with Positivity: Choose your environment and relationships wisely. Surround yourself with people who uplift and inspire you, who believe in your dreams, and who radiate positivity. Seek motivational books, podcasts, and uplifting content that nourishes your mind and spirit. Create a supportive ecosystem that fosters growth, resilience and a constant reminder of your potential.

7. Practice Self-Compassion: Be kind to yourself on this journey. Recognize that setbacks and challenges are a natural part of life. When faced with obstacles, practice self-

compassion and remind yourself that you are doing the best you can. Embrace vulnerability as an opportunity for growth and self-discovery. Treat yourself with the same love and understanding you would offer to a dear friend. By cultivating self-compassion, you fuel the flames of self-belief and resilience.

8. Cultivate a Growth Mindset: Embrace the mindset of continuous growth and learning. See failures as stepping stones to success, setbacks as opportunities for growth, and challenges as catalysts for transformation. Embrace the idea that you can always improve, evolve, and expand your capabilities. Embody the curiosity and resilience of a lifelong learner, and let your growth mindset fuel your pursuit of greatness.

9. Take Inspired Action: Let your positive mindset translate into action. Break down your goals into actionable steps and take consistent, intentional action toward their realization. Challenge yourself to step outside your comfort zone, embrace new opportunities, and push past your perceived limits. With each small step forward, you build momentum and stoke the fire of your inner flame.

10. Celebrate Your Victories: Along this journey of cultivating a positive mindset, remember to celebrate your victories, no matter how small. Acknowledge and appreciate the progress you have made, and let it inspire you to keep moving forward. Celebrate not only the destination but also the growth, resilience, and transformation you experience

along the way. Each milestone reached is a testament to the power of your positive mindset.

Now, take these action steps and let them become the fuel that ignites the flame within you. Embrace the power of your mindset, and let it guide you toward a life of boundless possibilities, resilience, and unwavering belief in your ability to create the life you desire. Together, let us embark on this transformative journey and set the stage for a future filled with success, joy, and fulfillment.

MY NOTES:

Chapter 4

Fueling Your Body:

Nourishment for Optimal Health and Vitality

Dear reader, as we embark on the fourth chapter of our transformative journey, let us delve into the realm of nourishment—a cornerstone of vibrant health and vitality. The food we consume is more than mere sustenance; it is the fuel that powers our bodies, minds, and souls.

In a world filled with endless dietary trends and conflicting information, it is crucial to navigate the sea of choices with wisdom and discernment. The key lies not in following strict rules or depriving ourselves but in embracing a holistic approach to nutrition—one that nourishes not only our physical bodies but also our emotional well-being.

At the heart of this chapter lies the understanding that food is not the enemy, but rather a source of healing, rejuvenation, and pleasure. We will explore the principles of mindful eating, honoring the body's signals of hunger and satiety, and cultivating a harmonious relationship with food.

Drawing inspiration from the groundbreaking works of renowned nutritionists and researchers, we will uncover the hidden dangers in certain foods and the transformative power of nutrient-dense choices. Books such as "The Plant Paradox," "The Obesity Code," and "Wheat Belly" have shed light on the detrimental effects of processed foods, refined sugars, and inflammatory ingredients. Armed with this knowledge, we can make informed choices that support our journey toward optimal health.

But let us not forget that nutrition is not solely about the physical aspects of our well-being. It is also deeply intertwined with our emotional connection to food. We will explore the role of emotional eating, the power of intuitive eating, and the importance of finding the balance between nourishment and enjoyment.

In the pages that follow, you will find practical guidance on creating a balanced, nutrient-rich diet that suits your unique needs and preferences. We will delve into the vibrant world of whole foods, embracing the bounty of nature and savoring the flavors and textures that nourish both body and soul.

Dear reader, as you embark on this chapter, let your emotions flow freely. Reflect on your relationship with food, your eating habits, and the choices you make daily. Explore the joy of preparing nourishing meals, the satisfaction of mindful eating, and the profound impact it can have on your overall well-being.

Take the time to experiment with new ingredients, flavors, and cooking techniques. Celebrate the abundance of nature and the gifts it provides. Let each meal become a moment of self-care, an opportunity to honor your body and nourish it from within.

At the end of this chapter, you will find practical tips, delicious recipes, and action steps to guide you on your path toward optimal nutrition. Remember, dear reader, the journey to the best shape of your life is not about perfection but progress. Embrace the power of nourishment, and let it fuel your body, mind, and spirit on the path to vibrant health and healthy life after 40.

Together, let us celebrate the transformative power of food and create a symphony of wellness, one bite at a time.

Actions to Take: Fuel Your Body for Optimal Health

1. Embrace the Power of Nourishment: Shift your perspective on food and embrace it as a powerful tool for nourishing your body, mind, and soul. Recognize that each meal is an opportunity to fuel your body with the nutrients it needs to thrive. Embrace the idea that food is not the enemy but a source of healing, rejuvenation, and pleasure.

2. Practice Mindful Eating: Engage in the practice of mindful eating. Slow down, savor each bite, and truly experience the flavors, textures, and aromas of your food. Pay attention to your body's hunger and satiety signals, allowing them to guide your eating habits. Be fully present in the moment, free from distractions, and cultivate a deep appreciation for the nourishment you receive.

3. Explore Nutrient-Dense Choices: Educate yourself about the transformative power of nutrient-dense foods. Discover the benefits of fresh fruits and vegetables, lean proteins, whole grains, and healthy fats. Experiment with incorporating a wide variety of colorful, plant-based foods into your diet. Embrace the concept of "eating the rainbow" to ensure you're getting a broad spectrum of essential vitamins, minerals, and antioxidants.

4. Navigate the Sea of Choices: In a world filled with dietary trends and conflicting information, approach food choices

with wisdom and discernment. Take the time to educate yourself about the potential risks and benefits of different foods. Be critical of marketing claims and rely on reputable sources of information to make informed decisions that align with your personal health goals.

5. Cultivate a Balanced Relationship with Food: Explore your emotional connection to food and cultivate a balanced relationship. Practice self-awareness and identify any patterns of emotional eating or restrictive behaviors. Nurture a mindset of nourishing your body while also allowing for enjoyment and occasional indulgences. Find the balance that works for you, where food is both a source of nourishment and a source of pleasure.

6. Experiment with New Ingredients and Recipes: Step out of your culinary comfort zone and experiment with new ingredients, flavors, and cooking techniques. Embrace the excitement of discovering new tastes and textures. Try out wholesome recipes that incorporate nutrient-dense foods, and let the creative process of cooking become a joyful and therapeutic experience.

7. Celebrate the Abundance of Nature: Develop a deep appreciation for the abundance of nature and the gifts it provides. Visit local farmers' markets, explore seasonal produce, and connect with the origins of your food. Celebrate the vibrant colors, fragrances, and flavors that nature offers. Let each meal become a celebration of the

earth's bounty and a reminder of our interconnectedness with the natural world.

8. Practice Meal Planning and Preparation: Take a proactive approach to your nutrition by engaging in meal planning and preparation. Set aside dedicated time each week to plan nutritious meals and prepare ingredients in advance. This will empower you to make healthier choices and avoid relying on processed or convenience foods during busy times. Meal planning also allows you to infuse your meals with love and intention, making them a reflection of self-care and nourishment.

9. Share the Joy of Nourishment: Invite loved ones to join you on this journey of nourishment. Share delicious meals and meaningful conversations around the table. Create a sense of community and connection through the act of nourishing both body and soul together. Let the joy of shared meals become a source of inspiration and motivation on your path to optimal health.

10. Embrace Progress, Not Perfection: Remember, dear reader, that the journey to optimal nutrition is not about perfection but progress. Embrace the power of nourishment and make small, sustainable changes that align with your individual needs and goals. Celebrate each step forward, no matter how small, and let the positive impact of nourishing your body ripple into all areas of your life.

Together, let us celebrate the transformative power of food and create a symphony of wellness, one bite at a time. Fuel your body with love, mindfulness, and nourishing choices, and experience the profound impact it has on your journey to vibrant health and healthy life after 40.

<u>**MY NOTES:**</u>

Chapter 5

Moving with Purpose:

Embracing the Joy of Physical Activity

Dear reader, as we embark on the fifth chapter of our transformative journey, let us delve into the realm of physical activity—a realm where the body and soul unite in a joyful dance of movement and vitality. It is within the rhythm of our steps, the power of our muscles, and the beating of our hearts that we find the key to unlocking our full potential.

In a world that often seduces us into a sedentary lifestyle, it is crucial to rediscover the joy and benefits of physical activity. Exercise is not merely a means to an end, but a gateway to a life of strength, resilience, and holistic well-being. It is a celebration of what our bodies are capable of, a testament to our innate power.

In this chapter, we will explore the profound impact of movement on our physical, mental, and emotional well-being. We will draw inspiration from books like "Younger Next Year" and "The 4-Hour Body," which emphasize the transformative power of exercise in maintaining youthful vigor and achieving extraordinary feats.

Let us redefine the notion of exercise as not just a chore, but a gift we give ourselves—a sacred time to honor our bodies and reconnect with our inner vitality. We will explore a wide range of activities, from cardiovascular exercises that strengthen our hearts to strength training that builds lean muscle mass and enhances our physical capabilities.

But beyond the physical benefits, physical activity is also a gateway to emotional release, stress reduction, and mental clarity. We will dive into the realm of mind-body practices such as yoga, tai chi, and meditation, which fuse movement with mindfulness, creating a harmonious union of body, mind, and spirit.

Dear reader, let your emotions soar as you embrace the joy of physical activity. Discover the activities that resonate with your soul, whether it be dancing, hiking, swimming, or practicing martial arts. Let each movement be a celebration of life, a testament to your commitment to be in the best shape of your life.

In the pages that follow, you will find practical guidance on incorporating physical activity into your daily routine. We will explore strategies for overcoming barriers and finding motivation when the road seems daunting. Through step-by-step instructions, actionable tips, and inspiring stories of transformation, you will be empowered to embark on a journey of movement and vitality.

Remember, dear reader, that the path to vibrant health is not about comparison or striving for perfection. It is about embracing the joy of movement, listening to your body's cues, and honoring your unique journey. Let each step, each breath, be an affirmation of your commitment to living a life filled with vitality and purpose.

At the end of this chapter, you will find practical action items and reflective exercises to guide you on your path to embracing the joy of physical activity. Take notes, set goals, and let each achievement become a stepping stone toward the best version of yourself.

Together, let us dance, run, stretch, and move with purpose. Let us create a symphony of strength, flexibility, and resilience that resonates throughout our lives. Embrace the transformative power of physical activity, and let it be the catalyst for a life of boundless energy, passion, and radiant health.

With each movement, let your emotions surge, let your spirit soar, and let your body revel in the joy of being alive.

Actions to Take: Embrace the Joy of Physical Activity

1. Redefine Exercise as Self-Care: Shift your perspective on physical activity and redefine it as an act of self-care and self-love. Embrace the idea that moving your body is a precious gift you give yourself—a time to honor and celebrate your innate power and vitality. Let go of the notion that exercise is a chore and embrace it as an opportunity to reconnect with the joy of movement.

2. Explore Activities that Resonate: Allow your emotions to guide you as you explore different activities that resonate with your soul. Whether it's dancing, hiking, swimming, or practicing martial arts, choose activities that bring you joy and make your heart sing. Let each movement be a celebration of life and an expression of your commitment to be in the best shape of your life.

3. Discover the Transformative Power: Recognize that physical activity extends beyond the physical realm. It is a gateway to emotional release, stress reduction, and mental clarity. Embrace mind-body practices like yoga, tai chi, or meditation that fuse movement with mindfulness, creating a harmonious union of body, mind, and spirit. Allow yourself to be fully present in each movement, experiencing the transformative power it holds.

4. Make Movement a Sacred Time: Carve out dedicated time for physical activity and make it a sacred ritual. Treat it as a time to honor your body, reconnect with your inner vitality, and prioritize your well-being. Create a supportive environment that encourages you to fully engage in the joy of movement without distractions. Let each session be a precious gift you give yourself, a time to invest in your physical and emotional health.

5. Overcome Barriers and Find Motivation: Acknowledge that the road to embracing physical activity may have its challenges. Identify potential barriers and develop strategies to overcome them. Surround yourself with a supportive community, set achievable goals, and find sources of inspiration that resonate with you. Remind yourself of the countless benefits and the incredible feeling of accomplishment that comes from pushing past your limits.

6. Listen to Your Body: Practice active listening to your body's cues and honor its needs. Pay attention to any discomfort or signs of overexertion, adjusting your activities accordingly. Embrace rest and recovery as essential parts of your journey and understand that progress is made through a balance of pushing yourself and respecting your limits. Let your body guide you toward sustainable and fulfilling movement practices.

7. Set Goals and Track Progress: Set specific, measurable goals to guide your journey of physical activity. Whether it's increasing the number of steps you take each day, mastering

a new yoga pose, or completing a marathon, set milestones that inspire and motivate you. Track your progress, celebrate each achievement, and let your accomplishments fuel your commitment to ongoing growth.

8. Infuse Movement into Daily Life: Find opportunities to infuse movement into your daily life, even beyond dedicated exercise sessions. Take the stairs instead of the elevator, go for a walk during your lunch break, or engage in active hobbies that bring you joy. Embrace the idea of a dynamic lifestyle where movement becomes an integral part of your daily routine.

9. Inspire and Be Inspired: Share your journey of physical activity with others and inspire those around you. Share your achievements, challenges, and lessons learned. Be a source of encouragement and support for others on their path to embracing movement and vitality. Surround yourself with like-minded individuals who uplift and motivate you to keep pushing forward.

10. Let Your Spirit Soar: With each movement, let your emotions surge, let your spirit soar, and let your body revel in the joy of being alive. Embrace the transformative power of physical activity and let it be the catalyst for a life of boundless energy, passion, and radiant health. Dance, run, stretch, and move with purpose, creating a symphony of strength, flexibility, and resilience that resonates throughout your life. Embrace the joy of physical activity and let it empower you to live life to the fullest.

MY NOTES:

Chapter 6

Restoring Balance:

The Power of Rest and Recovery

As we enter the sixth chapter of our transformative journey, let us explore the profound significance of rest and recovery—a realm often overlooked but essential for our overall well-being. In a world that glorifies constant productivity and hustle, it is vital to understand the transformative power of finding balance and honoring the restorative nature of rest.

Rest is not a sign of weakness or laziness, but a vital component of self-care and nurturing our body, mind, and soul. It is in these moments of stillness that we replenish our energy, heal from the demands of life, and regain our equilibrium.

In this chapter, we will draw inspiration from books like "The Blue Zones" and "Becoming Ageless," which highlight the importance of restful practices in promoting longevity, vitality, and a sense of well-being. We will explore the profound impact of quality sleep, relaxation techniques, and stress management on our overall health.

Let your emotions settle into a state of calm as we embrace the power of rest and recovery. Reflect on your current lifestyle and the balance—or lack thereof—between activity and rest. Let go of the guilt associated with taking time for yourself and immerse yourself in the healing embrace of stillness.

We will delve into the realm of sleep hygiene, exploring strategies to optimize the quality and duration of your sleep. We will uncover the rejuvenating power of relaxation techniques such as meditation, deep breathing, and mindfulness, which offer respite from the demands of the external world and allow us to connect with our inner selves.

In the pages that follow, you will discover practical tips on creating a restful environment, establishing a bedtime routine, and managing stress effectively. You will explore the profound impact of rest on your physical, mental, and emotional well-being and learn to prioritize self-care as an integral part of your journey toward the best shape of your life.

Remember, dear reader, that true well-being is not solely about pushing yourself to the limit or striving for constant achievement. It is about finding harmony, embracing the ebb and flow of life, and nurturing your body and mind with the rest they deserve. Let each moment of rest be an act of self-love and an affirmation of your worthiness.

At the end of this chapter, you will find actionable steps, reflective exercises, and practical tools to guide you on your path to restoring balance in your life. Take notes, set intentions, and let each moment of rest and recovery become a sacred act of self-care.

Together, let us create a symphony of rest and rejuvenation, allowing ourselves to be replenished, restored, and reinvigorated. Embrace the transformative power of rest, and let it be the foundation upon which you build a life of vibrant health, resilience, and lasting well-being.

In the silence of rest, let your emotions find solace, your body find healing, and your spirit find renewal.

Actions to Take: Embrace the Power of Rest and Recovery

1. Redefine Rest as Self-Nurturing: Shift your perspective on rest and recovery, understanding that it is not a sign of weakness or laziness, but a vital act of self-nurturing and self-care. Let go of the societal pressure to be constantly productive and embrace the transformative power of finding balance. Recognize that by honoring your need for rest, you replenish your energy, promote healing, and restore your overall well-being.

2. Reflect on Your Lifestyle: Allow your emotions to settle into a state of calm as you reflect on your current lifestyle and the balance—or lack thereof—between activity and rest. Be honest with yourself and identify areas where you may be neglecting rest and recovery. Release any guilt associated with taking time for yourself and embrace the healing embrace of stillness.

3. Prioritize Quality Sleep: Delve into the realm of sleep hygiene and prioritize the quality and duration of your sleep. Create a restful environment that promotes relaxation and establishes a consistent bedtime routine. Embrace the rejuvenating power of a good night's sleep, understanding that it is during this time that your body repairs, restores, and prepares itself for the challenges ahead.

4. Explore Relaxation Techniques: Discover the transformative power of relaxation techniques such as meditation, deep breathing, and mindfulness. Immerse yourself in moments of calm and stillness, allowing yourself to disconnect from the demands of the external world and connect with your inner self. Let go of stress and tension as you embrace the serenity that comes from practicing these techniques.

5. Create a Restful Environment: Designate a space in your home or surroundings that promotes relaxation and rest. Declutter your surroundings, add soothing elements such as candles or soft lighting, and surround yourself with objects that bring you peace and tranquility. Transform this space into your sanctuary, a haven where you can retreat and find solace.

6. Manage Stress Effectively: Recognize the impact of stress on your overall well-being and develop strategies to manage it effectively. Explore techniques such as journaling, engaging in hobbies, spending time in nature, or seeking support from loved ones. Prioritize self-care activities that help you unwind, recharge, and find balance amidst life's challenges.

7. Embrace the Ebb and Flow of Life: Remember that true well-being is not solely about constant achievement or pushing yourself to the limit. It is about embracing the ebb and flow of life, recognizing that rest and recovery are essential components of a healthy and fulfilling journey.

Embrace the rhythm of rest and activity, allowing yourself to find harmony and nurture your body and mind with the rest they deserve.

8. Practice Self-Love: Let each moment of rest be an act of self-love and an affirmation of your worthiness. Release any guilt or self-judgment associated with taking time for yourself and fully embrace the importance of self-care. Recognize that by prioritizing rest and recovery, you are investing in your long-term well-being and enabling yourself to show up as your best self in all aspects of life.

9. Integrate Rest into Your Routine: Incorporate intentional moments of rest and recovery into your daily routine. Schedule breaks throughout the day to recharge, engage in activities that bring you joy and relaxation, and honor your need for downtime. Integrate restful practices into your lifestyle as a non-negotiable aspect of your overall health and well-being.

10. Nurture Yourself with Rest: In the silence of rest, allow your emotions to find solace, your body to find healing, and your spirit to find renewal. Embrace the transformative power of rest and let it be the foundation upon which you build a life of vibrant health, resilience, and lasting well-being. Together, let us create a symphony of rest and rejuvenation, allowing ourselves to be replenished, restored, and reinvigorated.

MY NOTES:

48

Chapter 7

Cultivating Inner Resilience:

Nurturing Your Mental and Emotional Well-Being

In this chapter, we will draw inspiration from books like "The Hormone Reset Diet" and "Grain Brain," which shed light on the intricate connection between our mental and physical well-being. We will explore strategies for managing stress, fostering a positive mindset, and cultivating emotional balance.

Dear reader, let your emotions flow as we delve into the realm of mental and emotional well-being. Reflect on your own experiences, the challenges you have faced, and the resilience you have already demonstrated. Embrace your inner strength and believe in your ability to navigate life's obstacles with resilience and grace.

We will explore the power of self-care practices such as journaling, gratitude, and self-compassion, which nurture our inner landscape and help us cultivate a positive mindset. We will also dive into the transformative potential of mindfulness and meditation, which allow us to develop a deeper sense of self-awareness, manage stress, and cultivate emotional balance.

In the pages that follow, you will find practical techniques, insightful exercises, and empowering strategies to nurture your mental and emotional well-being. You will discover the power of reframing your thoughts, embracing self-compassion, and fostering a resilient mindset that empowers you to overcome challenges and thrive.

Remember, dear reader, that resilience is not about avoiding difficult emotions or pretending that everything is perfect. It is about acknowledging and honoring your emotions, finding healthy ways to cope, and embracing the growth that comes from navigating life's trials.

At the end of this chapter, you will find actionable steps, reflective exercises, and tools to guide you on your path to cultivating inner resilience. Take notes, practice self-reflection, and let each moment of self-care become a powerful act of self-love.

Together, let us create a symphony of inner strength and emotional well-being, nurturing our minds and hearts to weather life's storms with grace and resilience. Embrace the transformative power of cultivating inner resilience, and let it be the anchor that keeps you grounded, hopeful, and empowered on your journey to the best shape of your life.

In the depths of your emotions, find the strength to rise, the courage to persevere, and the wisdom to embrace each moment as an opportunity for growth.

Actions to Take: Cultivating Inner Resilience

1. Embrace Your Emotional Journey: Acknowledge and honor your emotions, both positive and negative. Recognize that every emotion holds valuable information about your inner world. Allow yourself to feel deeply and use your emotions as a compass to guide your actions and decisions.

2. Practice Self-Reflection: Set aside regular time for self-reflection and introspection. Engage in journaling to clarify your thoughts, feelings, and experiences. Reflect on the challenges you have faced and the lessons you have learned. Use this self-reflection as an opportunity to cultivate self-awareness and deepen your understanding of yourself.

3. Foster a Positive Mindset: Consciously choose to focus on the positive aspects of your life. Cultivate gratitude by acknowledging and appreciating the blessings, big and small, that surround you. Shift your perspective from problems to possibilities, and from obstacles to opportunities. Nurture a positive mindset that empowers you to approach life with optimism and resilience.

4. Practice Self-Compassion: Be kind and compassionate toward yourself, especially during times of difficulty or failure. Treat yourself with the same care and understanding you would extend to a dear friend. Embrace self-compassion as a powerful tool for healing, self-acceptance,

and growth. Remember that self-compassion allows you to bounce back from setbacks and cultivate resilience.

5. Engage in Mindfulness and Meditation: Incorporate mindfulness and meditation practices into your daily routine. These practices help you develop present-moment awareness and cultivate a deep connection with your inner self. Through mindfulness and meditation, you can manage stress, enhance emotional balance, and gain clarity amidst the chaos of life. Commit to regular practice and let these moments of stillness nourish your mind and spirit.

6. Reframe Your Thoughts: Become aware of negative or self-limiting thoughts that may arise. Challenge these thoughts by consciously reframing them into more positive and empowering perspectives. Cultivate a growth mindset that sees failures as opportunities for learning and setbacks as stepping stones toward success. Embrace the power of positive affirmations and choose thoughts that uplift and motivate you.

7. Seek Support and Connection: Recognize the importance of social connections and seek support from loved ones, friends, or support groups. Surround yourself with positive and supportive individuals who uplift and inspire you. Engage in meaningful conversations, share your experiences, and lean on others when needed. Remember that resilience is built not in isolation but through the support and connection we find in the community.

8. Take Care of Your Physical Well-Being: Nurture your mental and emotional well-being by taking care of your physical health. Engage in regular exercise, eat nourishing foods, and prioritize restful sleep. Remember that your mind and body are interconnected, and by caring for your physical well-being, you provide a solid foundation for cultivating inner resilience.

9. Embrace Vulnerability and Growth: Be willing to step outside your comfort zone and embrace vulnerability as a catalyst for personal growth. Recognize that it is through challenges and stretching your limits that you discover your true strength and resilience. Embrace the unknown with curiosity and openness, knowing that every step you take is an opportunity to grow and become the best version of yourself.

10. Take Action, One Step at a Time: Commit to taking small, actionable steps toward nurturing your mental and emotional well-being. Implement the strategies and exercises you discover in this chapter, and integrate them into your daily life. Remember that resilience is not built overnight but through consistent effort and dedication. Celebrate your progress along the way and trust in your ability to navigate life's challenges with resilience, grace, and unwavering determination.

Dear reader, let these "Take Action" sections serve as a roadmap to cultivate inner resilience and nurture your mental and emotional well-being. Trust in your capacity to embrace challenges, learn from setbacks, and emerge stronger than before. Your journey to the best shape of your life begins with the power of your thoughts, the kindness you show yourself, and the actions you take each day.

MY NOTES:

Chapter 8

Nourishing Your Body, Nourishing Your Soul:

The Power of Nutrition

Dear reader, as we enter the eighth chapter of our transformative journey, let us explore the profound connection between nourishing our bodies and nurturing our souls. In a world filled with processed foods and conflicting dietary advice, it is crucial to rediscover the transformative power of nutrition in promoting our overall well-being.

Food is not just fuel for our bodies; it is a source of nourishment, vitality, and connection. It is a language through which we express our love for ourselves and others. The choices we make when it comes to nourishing our bodies have a profound impact on our physical health, mental clarity, and emotional well-being.

In this chapter, we will draw inspiration from books like "The Plant Paradox" and "Wheat Belly," which shed light on the hidden dangers of certain foods and advocate for a more mindful approach to nutrition. We will explore the power of whole foods, the benefits of mindful eating, and the impact of nutrition on our energy levels, weight management, and long-term health.

Dear reader, let your emotions awaken as we delve into the realm of nutrition. Reflect on your relationship with food, the choices you make, and the impact they have on your overall well-being. Embrace the power of mindful eating, and let it be a gateway to a deeper connection with yourself and the nourishing qualities of food.

We will explore the importance of a balanced diet, rich in whole grains, lean proteins, healthy fats, and an abundance of fruits and vegetables. We will uncover the hidden dangers of processed foods, sugar, and artificial additives, and learn to make informed choices that support our health and vitality.

In the pages that follow, you will find practical guidance, delicious recipes, and insightful tips to help you make nourishing choices every day. We will explore the power of meal planning, mindful eating practices, and intuitive eating, which allow us to reconnect with our body's wisdom and find joy in the nourishment we provide.

Remember, dear reader, that nutrition is not about restrictive diets or perfection. It is about cultivating a healthy relationship with food, embracing a variety of nourishing choices, and savoring each bite with gratitude. Let each meal be an opportunity to fuel your body, nurture your soul, and honor the amazing vessel that carries you through life.

At the end of this chapter, you will find actionable steps, reflective exercises, and practical tools to guide you on your path to nourishing your body and soul. Take notes, experiment with new recipes, and let each food choice become an act of self-care and self-love.

Together, let us create a symphony of nourishment, celebrating the vibrant flavors, colors, and textures that nature provides. Embrace the transformative power of nutrition, and let it be the cornerstone of your journey to the best shape of your life—physically, mentally, and emotionally.

In nurturing your body, let your emotions bloom, your vitality soar, and you find solace.

Actions to Take: Nourishing Your Body, Nourishing Your Soul

1. Cultivate Mindful Eating: Practice mindful eating by bringing awareness and intention to your meals. Slow down, savor each bite, and pay attention to the flavors, textures, and sensations of the food. Engage your senses and fully immerse yourself in the present moment. Let mindful eating be a gateway to a deeper connection with your body and the nourishing qualities of food.

2. Embrace Whole Foods: Make a conscious effort to include a wide variety of whole foods in your diet. Incorporate an abundance of colorful fruits and vegetables, whole grains, lean proteins, and healthy fats. Opt for unprocessed and minimally processed foods whenever possible, as they provide essential nutrients and support your overall well-being.

3. Prioritize Meal Planning: Set aside time each week to plan your meals and snacks. Create a balanced menu that includes a variety of nutrient-dense foods. Meal planning not only helps you make healthier choices but also saves time and reduces stress in your day-to-day life. Experiment with new recipes and ingredients, and make nourishing meals a joyful part of your routine.

4. Connect with the Source of Your Food: Develop a deeper connection with the food you consume by understanding

its source. Learn about sustainable farming practices, support local farmers and markets, or even consider growing your herbs or vegetables. By appreciating the journey from farm to table, you can develop a greater appreciation for the nourishment provided by the earth.

5. Practice Intuitive Eating: Listen to your body's cues and honor its needs through intuitive eating. Pay attention to your hunger and fullness levels, and eat when you are physically hungry rather than based on external factors. Cultivate a non-judgmental attitude towards food and your body, allowing yourself to enjoy a wide range of foods in moderation while respecting your unique nutritional requirements.

6. Hydrate with Intent: Prioritize hydration as an essential part of nourishing your body and soul. Drink plenty of water throughout the day to support proper bodily functions and overall well-being. Infuse your water with fresh fruits, herbs, or even a splash of citrus to add flavor and make hydration a delightful experience.

7. Find Joy in Cooking: Rediscover the joy of cooking by experimenting with new recipes and flavors. Explore different cuisines, try new cooking techniques, and involve loved ones in the process. Cooking can be a creative and meditative practice that nourishes not only your body but also your soul. Embrace the transformative power of preparing nourishing meals with love and intention.

8. Practice Gratitude for Nourishment: Cultivate gratitude for the nourishment you receive from food. Before each meal, take a moment to express gratitude for the farmers, producers, and all those involved in bringing food to your plate. Acknowledge the nourishment and energy the food provides, and let gratitude infuse your eating experience with a sense of appreciation and abundance.

9. Listen to Your Body's Wisdom: Tune in to the signals your body sends you regarding food choices and portion sizes. Pay attention to how different foods make you feel physically, mentally, and emotionally. Develop a deeper understanding of your unique nutritional needs and make choices that support your overall well-being. Trust in your body's wisdom and let it guide your nourishment journey.

10. Share the Joy of Nourishment: Nourishment is not only an individual experience but also a means of connection and celebration. Share meals with loved ones, engage in meaningful conversations, and create memories around the table. Embrace the joy of nourishing others and let the act of sharing food deepen your bonds and nurture your soul.

Let these "Actions to Take" sections empower you to embrace the transformative power of nutrition and the joy of nourishing your body and soul. May your food choices be guided by mindfulness, gratitude, and a deep understanding of the connection between what you eat and how you feel. Embrace the nourishment that comes from within and let it radiate outward, empowering you to live a vibrant and fulfilling life.

MY NOTES:

Chapter 9

Unlocking Longevity Secrets: Lessons from the World's Healthiest Communities

Welcome to Chapter 9, dear reader, where we embark on a fascinating journey to unlock the secrets of longevity from the world's healthiest communities. These extraordinary places, known as Blue Zones, hold the key to not just living longer, but also thriving with vitality and purpose. Prepare to be inspired, motivated, and empowered as we explore the wisdom of these remarkable communities and learn how to apply their lessons to our own lives.

Imagine stepping into a world where age is just a number, where laughter and joy fill the air, and wisdom is cherished. In the Blue Zones, such as Okinawa in Japan, Sardinia in Italy, Nicoya in Costa Rica, Icaria in Greece, and Loma Linda in California, people not only live longer but also enjoy robust health well into their golden years. These communities have captured the attention of researchers and health enthusiasts alike and for good reason.

So, what makes these places so special? Is it their genes, their diet, or their lifestyle? The truth is, it's a combination of all these factors and more. The Blue Zones have created an environment that nurtures healthy habits and fosters a sense of purpose, which in turn supports longevity.

Let's begin with their dietary habits, inspired by "The Plant Paradox." Inhabitants of the Blue Zones consume a primarily plant-based diet, rich in fruits, vegetables, whole grains, and legumes. Their plates are filled with an array of colorful, nutrient-rich foods that provide the building blocks for a healthy body. But it's not just what they eat that matters—it's also how they eat. Meals are shared with loved ones, creating a sense of community and connection that nourishes both the body and the soul.

Physical activity is another cornerstone of their lifestyle, as highlighted by "Younger Next Year." Unlike the sedentary lifestyles that have become the norm in many modern societies, the people in Blue Zones engage in regular, natural movement. They walk, bike, garden, and perform daily tasks that keep their bodies active and strong. Exercise is not seen as a chore but as a natural part of their everyday lives.

But longevity goes beyond the physical aspects. These communities also prioritize social connections and a sense of purpose, which contribute to their overall well-being. "The Blue Zones," sheds light on the importance of social connections and community support. Inhabitants of Blue Zones have strong support networks and deeply rooted relationships. They find joy in simple pleasures, laughter, and spending quality time with loved ones. They also engage in activities that give them a sense of purpose and fulfillment, whether it's tending to their gardens, volunteering, or pursuing creative endeavors.

As we explore the secrets of these remarkable communities, let's remember that their lessons are not exclusive to them alone. We can incorporate these principles into our own lives and unlock the doors to a healthier, happier, and more fulfilling future.

Actions to Take: Unlocking Longevity Secrets

1. Fill your plate with vibrant, nutrient-rich foods: Embrace a plant-based diet, incorporating plenty of fruits, vegetables, whole grains, and legumes into your meals. These foods provide essential nutrients and antioxidants that promote health and longevity.

2. Share meals with loved ones: Cultivate a sense of community and connection by sharing meals with family and friends. This practice not only enhances the enjoyment of food but also fosters stronger relationships and emotional well-being.

3. Engage in regular, natural movement: Incorporate physical activity into your daily routine. Take walks, ride a bike, or find enjoyable ways to keep your body active. Aim for at least 30 minutes of moderate-intensity exercise most days of the week.

4. Find joy in purposeful activities: Discover activities that give you a sense of purpose and fulfillment. Volunteer for a cause you're passionate about, pursue creative hobbies or engage in projects that align with your values.

5. Cultivate social connections: Nurture your relationships and build a strong support network. Spend quality time with loved ones, join clubs or community groups, and seek opportunities to connect with others who share your interests.

6. Prioritize self-care: Make self-care a priority in your life. Engage in activities that promote relaxation, reduce stress, and enhance your well-being. This can include meditation, yoga, reading, or indulging in your favorite hobbies.

7. Discover your sense of purpose: Reflect on what brings you joy and fulfillment. Identify your passions, interests, and values, and align your life with them. Pursue activities that bring meaning to your life and allow you to make a positive impact on others.

8. Embrace the power of laughter: Find joy and humor in everyday life. Laughing not only uplifts your mood but also has numerous health benefits, including stress reduction and improved immune function.

9. Practice gratitude: Cultivate an attitude of gratitude by acknowledging and appreciating the blessings in your life. Take time each day to reflect on the things you are grateful for, big or small.

10. Surround yourself with positivity: Seek out positive influences in your environment. Surround yourself with supportive and uplifting people, read inspiring books, listen to uplifting music, and expose yourself to positive and motivating content.

By taking these actions, dear reader, you are setting yourself on a path to unlock the longevity secrets of the world's healthiest communities. Embrace these practices with an open heart and mind, and watch as your life transforms, allowing you to thrive beyond 40 with vitality, joy, and purpose.

MY NOTES:

Beyond Diets:

Embracing Sustainable Lifestyle Changes

Welcome to Chapter 10, dear reader, where we embark on an exciting journey beyond diets and delve into the transformative power of embracing sustainable lifestyle changes. Get ready to be captivated by a wealth of knowledge that will nourish your mind, invigorate your spirit, and empower you to create lasting, positive transformations. This chapter, guided by the wisdom of renowned experts and authors, will inspire you to reimagine the way you approach nutrition and embrace a sustainable, enjoyable path to a healthier lifestyle.

In a world where diets dominate the conversation, it's time to shift our focus from restrictive eating to the art of nourishment. Drawing from the insights of "Younger Next Year," and "The Plant Paradox," we will explore the importance of understanding food as a source of vitality and pleasure. It's time to unlock the secrets of a sustainable, enjoyable approach to nutrition that will propel you toward vibrant health, happiness, and longevity.

Picture a life where you no longer feel imprisoned by calorie counts or rigid meal plans. Imagine savoring each bite, embracing the abundance of flavors and textures, and discovering the joy of nourishing your body with whole, nutrient-dense foods. The time has come to free ourselves from the clutches of restrictive diets and instead embark on a lifelong journey of culinary exploration, rooted in sound nutrition principles.

Now, dear reader, let's dive into the transformative world of nutrition and explore the following key aspects that will guide you toward embracing sustainable lifestyle changes:

The Power of Whole, Nutrient-Dense Foods: Inspired by the insightful work of "The Plant Paradox," we will discover the magic of whole, nutrient-dense foods. These are the foods that nature provides in their unprocessed form—vibrant fruits, colorful vegetables, wholesome grains, and nourishing legumes. Embrace the abundance of plant-based goodness and delight in the immense nutritional benefits they offer. Fill your plate with a rainbow of colors, allowing each meal to be a celebration of vitality and well-being.

Learning to Eat Healthily: Navigating the vast landscape of nutrition can be overwhelming, but fear not, for you are not alone on this journey. I am here to guide you. Drawing from the wisdom of various authors and experts, we will delve into the principles of healthy eating. Learn how to create balanced meals that include lean proteins, healthy fats, and a variety of plant-based foods. Discover the importance of portion control and mindful eating, allowing you to truly savor each mouthful and develop a harmonious relationship with food.

Making Nutrition Fun and Exciting: Good nutrition doesn't have to be bland or boring. In fact, it can be a thrilling adventure that tickles your taste buds and ignites your creativity. Inspired by the innovative approaches of the author of "The Whole30," we will explore how to make nutrition an enjoyable and sustainable part of your life. Experiment with new flavors, try different cooking techniques, and embrace the sheer joy of preparing wholesome meals that nourish both your body and soul.

Embracing Mindful Eating: In our fast-paced world, mindful eating is a powerful practice that allows us to reconnect with our bodies and the food we consume. Inspired by the work of the authors of "Younger Next Year," we will delve into the art of mindful eating. Slow down, savor each bite, and pay attention to your body's hunger and fullness cues. Engage your senses and relish the textures, aromas, and flavors of the food on your plate. By practicing mindful eating, you can cultivate a deep appreciation for the nourishment that food provides, fostering a positive relationship with eating that goes beyond diets and restrictions.

Building a Foundation of Nutritional Knowledge: To embrace sustainable lifestyle changes, it's crucial to build a solid foundation of nutritional knowledge. Learn about the impact of carbohydrates, the benefits of healthy fats, and the significance of balancing macronutrients in your diet. Arm yourself with the knowledge to make informed choices and optimize your nutrition for long-term health and well-being.

Cultivating a Healthy Relationship with Food: Food is not just fuel for our bodies; it is also a source of pleasure, culture, and connection. In our quest for sustainable lifestyle changes, it's essential to cultivate a healthy relationship with food. Inspired by the insights of various authors, we will explore strategies to overcome emotional eating, develop a positive body image, and practice self-compassion. Let go of guilt and shame surrounding food choices, and instead, embrace a balanced approach that allows you to enjoy a wide array of foods while nourishing your body and honoring your well-being.

Discovering the Joy of Cooking: Cooking your meals can be a transformative experience that connects you to the ingredients, flavors, and traditions of different cultures. We will celebrate the joy of cooking. Experiment with new recipes, explore diverse cuisines and unleash your inner chef. Transform your kitchen into a place of creativity and self-expression, where you can whip up nourishing meals that are both delicious and aligned with your nutritional goals.

Seeking Support and Accountability: Embarking on a journey towards sustainable lifestyle changes is easier when you have support and accountability. Seek out a community of like-minded individuals who share your passion for healthy living. Engage in conversations, share experiences, and support one another on your quest for long-lasting health and well-being. Consider enlisting the help of a nutritionist or dietitian who can provide personalized guidance and ensure you stay on track toward your goals.

Dear reader, as we conclude this transformative chapter, let us celebrate the power we hold within ourselves to embrace a sustainable, enjoyable approach to nutrition. By unlocking the secrets of whole, nutrient-dense foods, learning to eat healthily with joy and creativity, and fostering a positive relationship with food, we can embark on a lifelong journey of vitality, balance, and radiant well-being. Let the nourishment of your body be a celebration of life, and let the joy of sustainable nutrition guide you towards thriving beyond 40 and beyond.

Actions to Take: Beyond Diets

1. Rediscover the Joy of Whole Foods: Embrace the vibrant colors and flavors of whole, nutrient-dense foods. Fill your shopping cart with fresh fruits, vegetables, lean proteins, and whole grains. Let these wholesome ingredients be the foundation of your meals, providing essential nutrients and nourishing your body.

2. Prioritize Balanced Meals: Create balanced meals that include a variety of macronutrients. Include lean proteins like chicken, fish, tofu, or legumes, paired with a colorful array of vegetables and a serving of whole grains or healthy fats. Balancing your meals helps sustain energy levels and supports overall well-being.

3. Practice Mindful Eating: Slow down, savor each bite, and listen to your body's hunger and fullness cues. Engage your senses, appreciate the textures and flavors, and cultivate a deeper connection with your meals. Mindful eating brings awareness to your eating habits and promotes a healthier relationship with food.

4. Expand Your Culinary Horizons: Step out of your comfort zone and explore new recipes, ingredients, and flavors. Experiment with international cuisines, spices, and herbs. Embrace the joy of cooking and discover the pleasure of preparing nourishing meals that excite your taste buds and fuel your body.

5. Cultivate a Supportive Food Environment: Create an environment that supports healthy eating choices. Keep your pantry stocked with nutritious options and minimize the presence of processed foods. Organize your kitchen for ease of meal preparation and invest in kitchen tools that make cooking enjoyable and efficient.

6. Stay Hydrated: Hydration is key to overall health and vitality. Make it a habit to drink plenty of water throughout the day. Carry a reusable water bottle with you as a reminder to stay hydrated and make water your beverage of choice.

7. Embrace the Power of Meal Prep: Spend some time each week planning and preparing your meals in advance. This saves time and ensures you have nutritious options readily available. Set aside a specific day to batch cook, portion meals, and store them for easy grab-and-go options during busy days.

8. Seek Knowledge and Resources: Continuously educate yourself about nutrition and wellness. Read books, follow reputable nutrition blogs, and consult with registered dietitians or nutritionists. Stay informed about the latest research and evidence-based practices to make well-informed choices for your health.

9. Engage in Mindful Grocery Shopping: Approach grocery shopping with intention and mindfulness. Make a list before you go, focusing on nutrient-dense foods. Stick to the perimeter of the store where fresh produce, lean proteins,

and dairy products are usually located. Avoid impulsive purchases by shopping with a purpose.

10. Practice Self-Compassion: Remember that sustainable lifestyle changes take time and effort. Be patient and kind to yourself throughout this journey. Celebrate your progress, embrace setbacks as opportunities for growth, and appreciate the positive changes you are making in your life. Nourishing your body with love and compassion is just as important as the food you eat.

Remember, you have the power to transform your relationship with food and embrace a sustainable, enjoyable approach to nutrition. By prioritizing whole, nutrient-dense foods, practicing mindfulness, expanding your culinary horizons, and cultivating a supportive environment, you are paving the way for long-lasting well-being.

MY NOTES:

Chapter 11

Cultivating Meaningful Connections:

The Power of Relationships in Your Journey

Dear reader, as we embark on the eleventh chapter of our transformative journey, let us explore the profound significance of cultivating meaningful connections and nurturing relationships in our pursuit of a healthy and fulfilling life. In a world that often emphasizes individual success and independence, it is crucial to recognize the immense power that lies within our connections with others.

Relationships are not mere transactions or fleeting interactions; they are the threads that weave the fabric of our existence. They have the power to uplift our spirits, bring joy to our hearts, and provide a sense of belonging and support. It is through meaningful connections that we find solace, encouragement, and a profound understanding of ourselves and others.

In this chapter, we will draw inspiration from books like "The Blue Zones" and "Becoming Ageless," which illuminate the importance of social connections in promoting longevity, happiness, and overall well-being. We will explore the various dimensions of relationships, from family and friendships to community and romantic partnerships, and discover the transformative power they hold.

Let your emotions blossom as we delve into the realm of relationships. Reflect on the quality of your connections, the depth of your bonds, and the impact they have on your overall well-being. Embrace the power of meaningful relationships, and let them be a source of strength, inspiration, and unconditional love.

We will explore the importance of communication, empathy, and active listening in fostering healthy relationships. We will delve into the transformative potential of forgiveness, compassion, and gratitude, which allow us to nurture deeper connections and cultivate an environment of love and support.

In the pages that follow, you will find practical guidance, reflective exercises, and empowering strategies to help you cultivate meaningful connections in your life. We will explore the art of effective communication, the power of vulnerability, and the beauty of authentic connection. Let each interaction be an opportunity to create a ripple of positivity and deepen your bonds with others.

Remember, dear reader, that relationships require effort, understanding, and a willingness to invest your time and energy. They are a reflection of the love and care you have for yourself and those around you. Let each connection be an act of kindness and a testament to the power of human connection.

At the end of this chapter, you will find actionable steps, reflective exercises, and practical tools to guide you on your path to cultivating meaningful connections. Take notes, reach out to loved ones, and let each relationship be a transformative experience that nourishes your soul, ignites your passions, and brings immense joy to your life.

Together, let us create a symphony of love, compassion, and authentic connection, celebrating the profound impact relationships have on our well-being. Embrace the transformative power of cultivating meaningful connections, and let them be the tapestry that enriches your journey to the best shape of your life—physically, mentally, and emotionally.

In the embrace of meaningful connections, let your emotions flourish, your heart find solace, and your soul find profound fulfillment.

Actions to Take: Cultivating Meaningful Connections

1. Prioritize Quality Time: Make a conscious effort to spend quality time with your loved ones. Create opportunities for shared experiences, meaningful conversations, and heartfelt connections. Dedicate uninterrupted time to truly engage and be present with the people who matter most in your life.

2. Practice Active Listening: Develop the skill of active listening in your relationships. Give others your full attention, maintain eye contact, and show genuine interest in their thoughts and feelings. Practice empathy and seek to understand their perspective, fostering deeper connections and nurturing a sense of trust and openness.

3. Express Appreciation: Regularly express gratitude and appreciation for the people in your life. Take a moment to acknowledge their contributions, express admiration for their qualities, and highlight the impact they have on your well-being. Small gestures of appreciation can strengthen bonds and create a positive atmosphere in your relationships.

4. Foster Open Communication: Encourage open and honest communication within your relationships. Create a safe space where everyone feels comfortable expressing their thoughts, emotions, and needs. Practice effective

communication skills, such as using "I" statements, active listening, and offering constructive feedback, to foster understanding and resolve conflicts.

5. Nurture Empathy and Compassion: Cultivate empathy and compassion in your interactions with others. Seek to understand their experiences, validate their feelings, and offer support and understanding. Practice acts of kindness and compassion, knowing that they have the power to transform relationships and create a sense of connection and belonging.

6. Show Up and Be Present: Be fully present in your relationships. Show up with authenticity, vulnerability, and a genuine desire to connect. Put away distractions, such as electronic devices, and give your undivided attention to the person in front of you. Practice active engagement and let your loved ones feel seen, heard, and valued.

7. Practice Forgiveness and Letting Go: Embrace forgiveness as a means of healing and strengthening your relationships. Release resentment and grudges, and choose to let go of past hurts. Practice compassion towards yourself and others, recognizing that forgiveness is a powerful tool for personal growth, reconciliation, and deepening connections.

8. Cultivate Shared Interests and Activities: Explore shared interests and engage in activities together. Find common hobbies, pursue adventures, or join community groups that

align with your passions. These shared experiences create bonds, foster a sense of belonging, and provide opportunities for joyful connections and cherished memories.

9. Be a Supportive Presence: Be a source of support and encouragement for the people in your life. Offer a listening ear, provide a helping hand, and celebrate their successes. Show up during challenging times and offer your love, empathy, and assistance. Being a supportive presence strengthens bonds and creates a sense of togetherness.

10. Cultivate Diverse Relationships: Embrace diversity in your relationships. Seek connections with individuals from different backgrounds, cultures, and perspectives. Embrace the richness of diverse experiences and learn from one another. By expanding your circle of connections, you open doors to new insights, personal growth, and a broader understanding of the world.

Let these "Actions to Take" sections inspire you to cultivate meaningful connections and nurture relationships in your life. May each interaction be an opportunity to create a ripple of positivity, deepen your bonds, and bring immense joy to your life. Embrace the transformative power of authentic connection and let it enrich your journey to the best shape of your life—physically, mentally, and emotionally. In the embrace of meaningful connections, may your emotions flourish, your heart finds solace, and your soul finds profound fulfillment.

MY NOTES:

Chapter 12

Mindful Living:

Enhancing Mental Well-being

As we enter the twelfth chapter of our transformative journey, let us explore the profound significance of mindful living in enhancing our mental well-being. In a fast-paced world that often pulls us in different directions, it is essential to cultivate a conscious and present way of being that nurtures our mental health and fosters inner peace.

Mindful living is not a fleeting trend or a temporary fix; it is a way of life—a practice that allows us to fully engage with the present moment, cultivate self-awareness, and build resilience in the face of life's challenges. It is through mindful living that we tap into the boundless wisdom within ourselves and find a deep connection to the world around us.

In this chapter, we will draw inspiration from books like "The Power of Now" and "Wherever You Go, There You Are," which illuminate the transformative power of mindfulness in promoting mental well-being, reducing stress, and increasing overall happiness. We will explore the different dimensions of mindful living and discover practical strategies to incorporate mindfulness into our daily lives.

Let your emotions settle as we delve into the realm of mindful living. Reflect on the pace of your life, the moments of presence you experience, and the impact they have on your mental well-being. Embrace the power of mindfulness, and let it be a guiding light that illuminates your path toward clarity, peace, and serenity.

Actions to Take: Enhancing Mental Well-Being

1. Cultivate Present-Moment Awareness: Practice being fully present in each moment. Notice the sensations in your body, the thoughts in your mind, and the emotions in your heart. Engage your senses and immerse yourself in the richness of the present moment. Embrace the beauty of what is happening right here, right now.

2. Practice Mindful Breathing: Develop a regular practice of mindful breathing. Set aside a few moments each day to focus your attention on the rhythm of your breath. Observe each inhale and exhale, allowing your breath to anchor you to the present moment. Notice how this simple act of conscious breathing can bring a sense of calm and clarity to your mind.

3. Engage in Mindful Eating: Bring mindfulness to your eating habits. Slow down, savor each bite, and fully engage your senses in the experience of nourishing your body. Pay attention to the flavors, textures, and aromas of your food. Cultivate gratitude for the nourishment it provides. Eating mindfully can enhance your connection to your body and promote a healthier relationship with food.

4. Create Mindful Rituals: Incorporate mindful rituals into your daily life. Whether it's a morning meditation, a gratitude journaling practice, or a mindful walk in nature, find activities that ground you in the present moment and

bring a sense of peace and intention to your day. These rituals serve as anchors that remind you to come back to the present and cultivate a mindful mindset.

5. Practice Self-Compassion: Nurture a kind and compassionate relationship with yourself. Cultivate self-acceptance and embrace your imperfections. When faced with challenges or setbacks, practice self-compassion by treating yourself with the same kindness and understanding you would offer a dear friend. Remember, you are deserving of love, care, and forgiveness.

6. Engage in Mindful Movement: Incorporate mindful movement into your routine. Whether it's yoga, tai chi, or simply taking a mindful walk, engage your body and mind in the present moment. Notice the sensations in your body, the rhythm of your breath, and the connection between movement and stillness. Allow the practice of mindful movement to bring balance and vitality to your life.

7. Practice Gratitude: Cultivate a gratitude practice to shift your focus to the positive aspects of life. Each day, take a moment to reflect on the things you are grateful for. It can be as simple as appreciating a beautiful sunset, a kind gesture from a loved one, or the comfort of a warm cup of tea. Gratitude cultivates a sense of abundance and contentment, promoting mental well-being.

8. Create Digital Boundaries: Establish healthy boundaries with technology and digital distractions. Set aside

designated times to disconnect from screens and engage in activities that promote mindfulness and connection. Create sacred spaces free from the constant noise of notifications, allowing yourself to recharge and find solace in the present moment.

9. Practice Loving-Kindness Meditation: Engage in loving-kindness meditation to cultivate compassion and empathy towards yourself and others. Set aside time each day to send kind wishes and well-being to yourself, your loved ones, and even those who may challenge you. This practice nurtures a sense of interconnectedness and fosters a more positive and compassionate outlook on life.

10. Seek Mindful Relationships: Surround yourself with individuals who value mindfulness and embrace a conscious way of living. Seek out relationships that support your growth, well-being, and mindfulness practice. Engage in meaningful conversations, deep listening, and authentic connections that foster mutual understanding and growth.

Let these actions guide you on your path to mindful living and enhancing your mental well-being. Embrace the transformative power of mindfulness and let it bring clarity, peace, and serenity to your life. In the embrace of mindful living, may your mind find stillness, your heart find balance, and your soul find profound fulfillment.

MY NOTES:

Chapter 13

Movement as Medicine:

Exploring the Benefits of Yoga and Meditation

In this chapter, we dive into the transformative power of movement as medicine, focusing specifically on the incredible benefits of yoga and meditation. These ancient practices have stood the test of time, offering holistic approaches to physical, mental, and emotional well-being. As we explore the profound impact that yoga and meditation can have on our lives, we invite you to embark on a journey of self-discovery, healing, and inner peace.

The Healing Power of Yoga:

We begin by delving into the healing power of yoga. Through the practice of asanas (poses), pranayama (breathing exercises), and meditation, yoga offers a holistic approach to wellness. We'll explore how yoga enhances flexibility, strength, balance, and posture while promoting relaxation, stress reduction, and mental clarity. Discover the immense benefits of incorporating yoga into your daily routine and tap into your body's innate wisdom.

Nurturing the Mind and Soul with Meditation:

Next, we delve into the transformative practice of meditation. By cultivating mindfulness and a deep connection with the present moment, meditation allows us to quiet the mind, reduce stress, and enhance overall well-being. We'll explore different meditation techniques, from focused attention to loving-kindness, and provide practical guidance on how to incorporate meditation into your daily life. Discover the profound impact that meditation can have on your mental and emotional well-being.

Integrating Yoga and Meditation into Your Life:

In this section, we explore practical ways to integrate yoga and meditation into your daily life. We'll discuss the importance of consistency, creating a sacred space for practice, and finding a balance between effort and surrender. Whether you're a beginner or an experienced practitioner, you'll find guidance on establishing a sustainable and nourishing yoga and meditation practice that supports your overall well-being.

Actions to Take: Movement as Medicine

1. Begin a Yoga Practice: Start your yoga journey by finding a local studio, joining a virtual class, or exploring online resources. Commit to practicing yoga regularly, even if it's just a few minutes each day. Embrace the physical and mental benefits of yoga as you cultivate strength, flexibility, and inner peace.

2. Explore Different Yoga Styles: Expand your horizons by exploring various yoga styles such as Hatha, Vinyasa, Kundalini, or Yin. Each style offers unique benefits and approaches to movement and meditation. Try different classes or online tutorials to find the style that resonates with you and supports your well-being.

3. Establish a Daily Meditation Practice: Set aside time each day for meditation. Start with just a few minutes and gradually increase the duration as you become more comfortable. Find a quiet space, sit comfortably, and focus on your breath, a mantra, or a guided meditation. Cultivate a regular meditation practice to calm the mind, reduce stress, and foster inner stillness.

4. Attend a Meditation Retreat: Immerse yourself in a meditation retreat to deepen your practice and connect with like-minded individuals. Retreats offer a supportive environment for self-reflection, growth, and rejuvenation. Explore retreat options in your area or consider virtual

retreats that allow you to participate from the comfort of your own home.

5. Practice Mindful Movement Outside of Yoga: Incorporate mindfulness into your everyday activities. Engage in mindful walking, mindful eating, or simply being fully present in your daily tasks. Cultivate awareness and appreciation for each moment, regardless of whether you're on the yoga mat or off.

6. Join a Yoga Community: Connect with a yoga community to find support and inspiration. Attend yoga workshops, join online forums, or participate in group classes. Engaging with a community of like-minded individuals will enhance your yoga and meditation journey and provide a sense of belonging and encouragement.

7. Deepen Your Understanding: Expand your knowledge by reading books, articles, and blogs on yoga and meditation. Educate yourself about the philosophy, history, and science behind these practices. Deepening your understanding will enrich your practice and provide a broader perspective on their transformative potential.

8. Experiment with Pranayama Techniques: Explore the powerful benefits of pranayama, or breathwork. Experiment with different techniques such as alternate nostril breathing, deep belly breathing, or kapalabhati. Pranayama techniques can help calm the mind, energize the body, and balance your overall energy.

9. Create a Sacred Space for Practice: Designate a specific area in your home as a sacred space for your yoga and meditation practice. Decorate it with meaningful items, such as candles, incense, or inspiring images. Make it a space that brings you a sense of peace, tranquility, and focus.

10. Embrace the Journey: Approach your yoga and meditation practice with curiosity, patience, and self-compassion. Embrace the ups and downs, the challenges and breakthroughs. Remember that it's a lifelong journey of self-discovery and growth. Allow yourself to evolve and be open to the transformative power of these practices in your life.

Dear reader, may these actions guide you on your journey of embracing yoga and meditation as transformative tools for physical, mental, and emotional well-being. Through consistent practice, openness, and self-reflection, you can tap into the healing power of movement and cultivate inner peace. In the embrace of yoga and meditation, may your body find strength, your mind find clarity, and your soul finds profound serenity.

MY NOTES:

Chapter 14

Transforming Habits:

Sustaining Positive Change

In this chapter, we embark on a journey of transformation by focusing on the power of habits. Our lives are shaped by the habits we cultivate, and by understanding the science behind habit formation, we can consciously design our habits to support positive change. Get ready to unleash your full potential as we delve into the strategies and techniques that will empower you to transform your habits and sustain long-lasting positive change.

The Science of Habit Formation:

We begin by exploring the science behind habit formation. Understanding the habit loop and the role of cues, routines, and rewards allows us to gain insight into how habits are created and maintained. We'll also explore the concept of habit stacking and how to leverage existing habits to create new ones. By diving deep into the science of habits, you'll gain the knowledge needed to reshape your behaviors and embrace positive change.

Designing Your Ideal Habits:

Next, we guide you through the process of designing your ideal habits. We'll help you identify the habits that align with your goals and values, and create a roadmap for implementing them into your daily life. Through introspection and self-reflection, you'll gain clarity on the habits you want to cultivate and the ones you want to leave behind. It's time to take control of your habits and create a foundation for sustained positive change.

Strategies for Habit Transformation:

In this section, we provide you with practical strategies to transform your habits. We'll explore techniques such as habit tracking, habit stacking, and habit substitution. You'll learn how to overcome obstacles, deal with setbacks, and stay motivated throughout your habit transformation journey. We'll also discuss the importance of self-compassion and celebrate small wins along the way. By implementing these strategies, you'll create a supportive environment for positive habits to thrive.

Nurturing Consistency and Accountability:

Consistency is key when it comes to sustaining positive change. In this section, we delve into the importance of accountability and how it can help you stay on track with your new habits. We'll explore different accountability methods, such as finding an accountability partner or joining a community of like-minded individuals. By nurturing consistency and accountability, you'll reinforce your commitment to positive change and increase the likelihood of long-term success.

Actions to Take: Transforming Habits

1. Reflect on Your Current Habits: Take time to reflect on your current habits and their impact on your life. Identify which habits align with your goals and values and which ones may be hindering your progress. Awareness is the first step toward transformation.

2. Set Clear Goals: Define clear goals that you want to achieve through habit transformation. Whether it's improving your health, enhancing productivity, or cultivating mindfulness, having specific goals will provide direction and motivation for changing your habits.

3. Start Small: Begin your habit transformation journey by starting small. Focus on one habit at a time to avoid feeling overwhelmed. By mastering one habit, you'll build confidence and momentum to tackle larger changes.

4. Create a Habit Implementation Plan: Develop a detailed plan for implementing your desired habits. Break them down into smaller steps, set reminders, and establish a timeline. Having a well-structured plan will increase the likelihood of success and help you stay on track.

5. Surround Yourself with Support: Seek support from friends, family, or a community of individuals who share similar goals. Share your habit transformation journey with them and ask for their encouragement and accountability.

Supportive relationships can motivate during challenging times.

6. Practice Mindfulness: Incorporate mindfulness into your daily routine. Pay attention to your thoughts, emotions, and actions as you work towards changing your habits. Mindfulness will help you develop a deeper understanding of your habits and empower you to make conscious choices.

7. Track Your Progress: Keep a record of your habit transformation progress. Use a habit tracker or journal to monitor your daily habits and track your achievements. Celebrate milestones and use setbacks as learning opportunities to refine your approach.

8. Practice Self-Compassion: Be kind to yourself throughout the habit transformation process. Acknowledge that change takes time and effort, and setbacks are a natural part of the journey. Treat yourself with compassion and maintain a positive mindset.

9. Find Joy in the Process: Embrace the joy of habit transformation by focusing on the positive aspects of your journey. Celebrate the small wins, savor the positive changes you experience, and find gratitude for the opportunity to grow and evolve.

10. Embrace Iteration and Adaptation: Recognize that habit transformation is an ongoing process. Be open to adjusting your approach, experimenting with different strategies, and

refining your habits along the way. Embrace the journey of continuous improvement and adapt as needed.

May these actions empower you to transform your habits and sustain positive change in your life. Remember, change begins with small steps, consistency, and self-compassion. Embrace the power of habit transformation and create a life that aligns with your goals and values. In the embrace of intentional habits, let your actions shape your destiny and lead you to a future of growth, fulfillment, and lasting positive change.

MY NOTES:

Chapter 15

Thriving Together:

Building a Supportive Community

In this chapter, we emphasize the power of community and the immense impact it can have on our health and well-being. Humans are inherently social beings, and building a supportive community is essential for personal growth, resilience, and happiness. Together, we'll explore the benefits of fostering connections, nurturing relationships, and finding your tribe. Get ready to thrive as we dive into the world of community and discover how it can elevate your life.

The Importance of Connection:

We begin by discussing the importance of connection and the profound effects it has on our mental, emotional, and physical well-being. We'll explore the science behind human connection and how it influences our overall health. From reducing stress and loneliness to boosting self-esteem and providing a sense of belonging, connection is a fundamental aspect of our well-being.

Nurturing Relationships:

Next, we delve into the art of nurturing relationships. We'll explore strategies for building strong and meaningful connections with others. From active listening and empathy to effective communication and conflict resolution, you'll learn practical tools for cultivating healthy and supportive relationships. Discover the joy and fulfillment that comes from fostering deep connections with like-minded individuals.

Finding Your Tribe:

In this section, we focus on finding your tribe—the community of people who share your values, interests, and aspirations. We'll guide you through the process of seeking out communities that align with your passions, whether it's through local meetup groups, online forums, or social media platforms. We'll explore the benefits of joining communities that resonate with your goals, whether it's a fitness group, a book club, or a volunteer organization. By finding your tribe, you'll surround yourself with individuals who uplift, inspire, and support you on your journey to optimal health and wellness.

Nurturing a Supportive Community:

In this section, we discuss the importance of actively contributing to and nurturing a supportive community. We'll explore ways to engage and participate in your chosen communities, whether it's through sharing knowledge, offering support, or organizing events. By being an active member, you not only contribute to the well-being of others but also create a network of support that will be there for you when you need it most.

Actions to Take: Building a Supportive Community

1. Reflect on Your Need for Connection: Take a moment to reflect on your need for connection and the impact it has on your overall well-being. Recognize that building a supportive community is not just a luxury but a fundamental aspect of human existence. Embrace the truth that we thrive when we are surrounded by people who love, support and inspire us.

2. Step Out of Your Comfort Zone: Challenge yourself to step out of your comfort zone and actively seek opportunities for connection. Attend social events, join clubs or organizations, and engage in activities that align with your interests. Embrace the discomfort that comes with new experiences and open yourself up to the possibility of forming meaningful connections.

3. Be Open and Authentic: Approach relationships with openness and authenticity. Allow yourself to be vulnerable and share your true self with others. By being genuine, you create a space for others to do the same, fostering deeper and more meaningful connections. Embrace the beauty of authenticity and let it be the foundation of your relationships.

4. Practice Active Listening: Cultivate the art of active listening in your interactions with others. Give your undivided attention, show genuine interest, and seek to

understand the perspectives and experiences of those around you. By being fully present in conversations, you demonstrate respect and create a sense of connection that goes beyond surface-level interactions.

5. Foster Empathy and Compassion: Develop empathy and compassion towards others. Seek to understand their challenges, struggles, and triumphs. Practice kindness and offer support when needed. By nurturing empathy and compassion, you create a safe and nurturing environment where individuals can thrive and feel understood.

6. Create Opportunities for Connection: Take the initiative to create opportunities for connection within your community. Organize events, gatherings, or group activities that bring people together. Foster a sense of belonging and create spaces where individuals can share their passions, interests, and aspirations. By being a catalyst for connection, you contribute to the growth and well-being of your community.

7. Celebrate Diversity and Inclusion: Embrace diversity and promote inclusivity within your community. Recognize and appreciate the unique strengths and perspectives that each individual brings. Create a space where everyone feels valued, respected, and heard. Celebrate the richness that comes from embracing diverse backgrounds, experiences, and identities.

8. Show Gratitude and Appreciation: Express gratitude and appreciation for the individuals who form your supportive community. Take the time to acknowledge their presence, kindness, and support. By expressing gratitude, you strengthen the bonds within your community and cultivate a culture of positivity and appreciation.

9. Be a Source of Support: Be a source of support for others within your community. Offer encouragement, lend a helping hand, and be a compassionate listener. By being there for others, you create a reciprocal cycle of support where everyone benefits and feels uplifted.

10. Embrace the Power of Connection: Embrace the transformative power of connection in your life. Recognize that building a supportive community is not just about receiving support but also about giving it. Embrace the joy, inspiration, and motivation that come from being part of a community that uplifts and empowers you. Let connection be the fuel that propels you toward personal growth, resilience, and happiness.

Dear reader, as you embark on the journey of building a supportive community, remember that you have the power to create a network of love, understanding, and inspiration. Embrace the connections that come your way, nurture them with authenticity and kindness, and watch as your life flourishes in the embrace of a thriving community. Together, let us build a world where everyone feels seen, heard, and supported, and let our collective strength and compassion create a ripple effect of positive change.

MY NOTES:

Conclusion

In conclusion, "Thriving Beyond 40: How to Achieve Optimal Health and Wellness for a Fulfilling Life" has been a transformative journey, empowering you to embrace positive changes and unlock your full potential. Throughout this book, we have explored the power of mindset, nutrition, fitness, self-care, and community in creating a vibrant and fulfilling life.

You have learned to cultivate a growth mindset, embracing the belief that it's never too late to make positive changes and achieve your goals. You have discovered the impact of nourishing your body with wholesome and nutritious foods, supporting your overall well-being. You have experienced the transformative effects of regular physical activity, creating strength, endurance, and vitality.

Self-care has become a cornerstone of your daily routine, allowing you to prioritize your mental, emotional, and physical well-being. You have embraced the power of mindfulness, meditation, and breathwork to find peace, reduce stress, and enhance your overall quality of life.

But the journey doesn't end here. As you continue to implement the knowledge and practices from this book, remember that true transformation requires ongoing dedication and commitment. Embrace the journey as a lifelong pursuit of optimal health and wellness.

Surround yourself with a supportive community that uplifts and inspires you. Share your knowledge, experiences, and successes with others, and continue to learn and grow from the wisdom of those around you. Together, we can create a ripple effect of positive change, not only in our own lives but also in the lives of those we touch.

Remember, age is just a number. With a positive mindset, nourishing habits, self-care practices, and a supportive community, you have the power to thrive at any stage of life. Embrace the possibilities, live with intention, and create a life that is vibrant, fulfilling, and meaningful.

You are the author of your own story. So go forth with confidence, resilience, and a burning passion for a life filled with health, happiness, and purpose. Thrive beyond 40 and beyond, for the possibilities are limitless. Embrace the wisdom you have gained from this book and let it guide you as you continue to navigate the path of optimal health and wellness.

Remember that setbacks and challenges may arise along the way, but they are opportunities for growth and learning. Embrace them as part of your journey and use them as stepping stones toward greater resilience and success.

Celebrate your progress, no matter how small, and acknowledge the positive changes you have made. Each step forward is a testament to your dedication and determination. Allow yourself to bask in the joy of your achievements and let them fuel your motivation to keep moving forward.

As you thrive in your own life, extend a helping hand to others who may be seeking guidance and support. Share the knowledge and insights you have gained from this book, and be a source of inspiration and encouragement for those around you. Together, we can create a ripple effect of positive change that reaches far beyond ourselves.

In closing, remember that the journey toward optimal health and wellness is a lifelong one. Embrace it with curiosity, passion, and an open heart. Continuously seek knowledge, explore new possibilities, and adapt your approach as needed.

You have the power to shape your destiny and live a life of vitality, purpose, and fulfillment. Believe in yourself, trust in your abilities, and know that you are capable of achieving extraordinary things.

Thank you for joining us on this transformative journey in "Thriving Beyond 40: How to Achieve Optimal Health and Wellness for a Fulfilling Life." May it serve as a constant source of inspiration, guidance, and empowerment as you embark on a life of thriving and continue to rewrite your own story.

Remember, the best is yet to come. Keep thriving, keep growing, and keep embracing the beauty and joy that life has to offer. Your future is bright, and you have all the tools you need to make it an extraordinary one.

Here's to a life filled with health, happiness, and boundless possibilities. Cheers to thriving beyond 40 and living a life of optimal health and wellness!

Much love,

J.C. Osorio

Research

"Younger Next Year: Live Strong, Fit, and Sexy - Until You're 80 and Beyond" by Chris Crowley and Henry S. Lodge, M.D.

"The Blue Zones: Lessons for Living Longer From the People Who've Lived the Longest" by Dan Buettner.

"The Plant Paradox: The Hidden Dangers in 'Healthy' Foods That Cause Disease and Weight Gain" by Steven R. Gundry, M.D.

"The Hormone Reset Diet: Heal Your Metabolism to Lose Up to 15 Pounds in 21 Days" by Sara Gottfried, M.D.

"The Obesity Code: Unlocking the Secrets of Weight Loss" by Jason Fung.

"Wheat Belly: Lose the Wheat, Lose the Weight, and Find Your Path Back to Health" by William Davis, M.D.

"The Whole30: The 30-Day Guide to Total Health and Food Freedom" by Melissa Hartwig Urban and Dallas Hartwig.

"Grain Brain: The Surprising Truth about Wheat, Carbs, and Sugar - Your Brain's Silent Killers" by David Perlmutter, M.D.

"The 4-Hour Body: An Uncommon Guide to Rapid Fat-Loss, Incredible Sex, and Becoming Superhuman" by Timothy Ferriss.

"Becoming Ageless: The Four Secrets to Looking and Feeling Younger Than Ever" by Strauss Zelnick.

Additional Materials, Resources, and Coaching

To learn more, visit:

www.foreveryoungcoachinngacademy.com